28 DAYS CHAIR YOGA CHALLENGE FOR SENIORS

28 DAYS GUIDE FOR YOU TO IMPROVE YOUR FLEXIBILITY, MOBILITY, BALANCE, RELIEF STRESS AND LOSE WEIGHT.

DONNIE MAVERICK

COPYRIGHT NOTICE
© DONNIE MAVERICK 2024

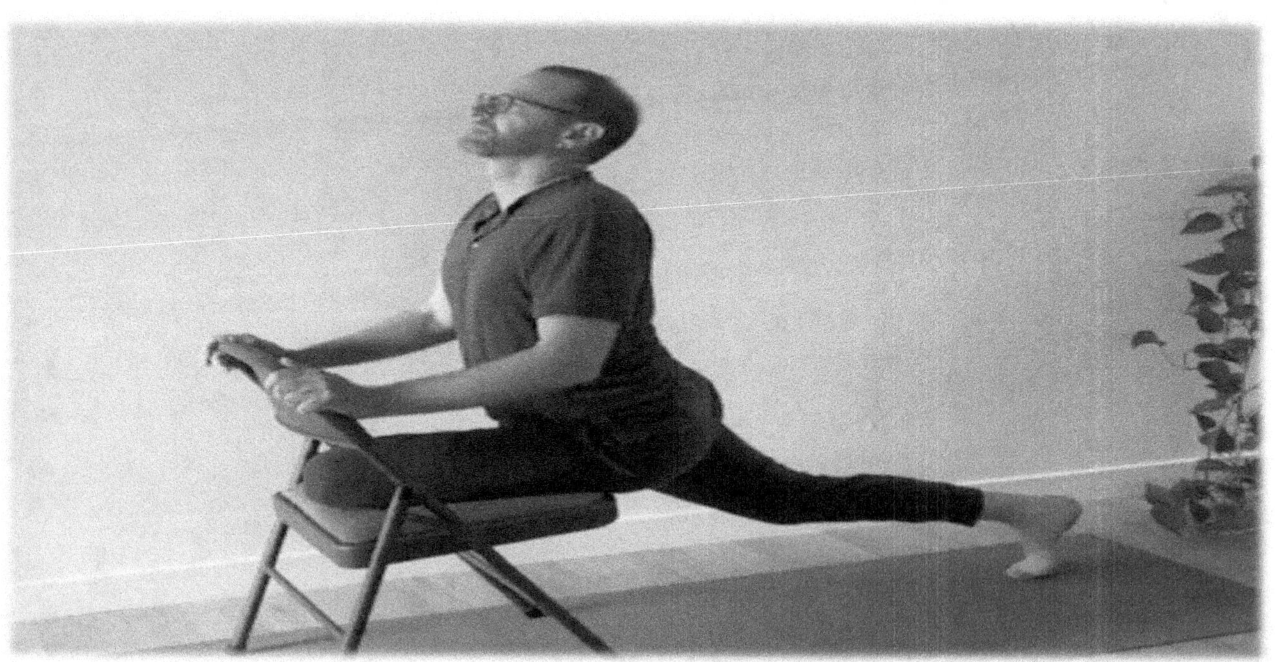

TABLE OF CONTENT

THIS BOOK OFFERS BROAD EXERCISE ON CHAIR YOGA.

AS A SENIOR THIS IS THE BOOK YOU NEED TO OVERCOME STRESS, GAIN BALANCE AND LOSE WEIGHT

INTRODUCTION

Welcome to the 28-Day Chair Yoga Challenge for Seniors, a transforming journey that brings the many benefits of yoga to the comfort of your chair. This thorough handbook is designed with seniors' special needs and considerations in mind, providing a gentle but effective approach to improving physical well-being, mental clarity, and emotional balance.

As we become older, keeping an active lifestyle becomes increasingly important for our general health. Chair yoga, a modified version of conventional yoga, emerges as an accessible and effective alternative for anyone looking to reap the full benefits of this ancient practice while adjusting to the demands of sitting activities.

This book is a guide to living a better, more balanced life, designed exclusively for seniors. Over the following 28 days, you will go on a varied trip that includes sitting exercises, mindful visualizations, and relaxation methods. Each day has a carefully chosen series of moves supported by comprehensive directions, allowing you to engage confidently and comfortably, regardless of your yoga experience or fitness level.

The exercises on these pages are intended to increase flexibility, balance, strength, and generate a sense of calm. The chair transforms into your own yoga mat, and each movement invites you to reconnect with your body, renew your mind, and enjoy the freedom of movement.

Remember that this is more than simply a routine; it is a comprehensive approach to wellness. Whether you're new to yoga or an experienced practitioner, the next 28 days are an opportunity to rediscover your extraordinary potential. So, sit comfortable in your chair, open your mind, and let us go on this empowering trip together. Your journey to better health and energy begins right now, with the 28 Days Chair Yoga Challenge for Seniors.

Laura, a senior, lived in a tranquil area surrounded by tall trees and singing birds. Despite her sweet nature, Evelyn suffered from the aches and pains that come with age. Determined to find comfort and renewal, she stumbled onto the 28 Days Chair Yoga Challenge for Seniors.

Evelyn set off on the voyage described in the book, skeptical but hopeful. Each morning, she sank into her favorite chair and followed the book's gentle motions and peaceful meditations.

As the days passed, Evelyn recognized small changes inside herself. Her joints' rigidity subsided, giving way to fresh flexibility and elegance. With each breath, she felt a sense of tranquility flood over her, as if the world's problems faded away.

Weeks progressed into months, and everyone who knew Evelyn saw her shift. Her laughter resonated louder, her feet were lighter, and her personality glowed with renewed vibrancy.

Evelyn felt not just physical comfort but also a deeper connection to herself and her surroundings thanks to the simple yet profound direction of the 28 Days Chair Yoga Challenge for Seniors. In the loving embrace of her chair, she discovered the strength to greet each day with appreciation and delight.

1. Gentle Exercise regimen: The 28 Days Chair Yoga for Seniors challenge includes a gentle exercise regimen created exclusively for the elderly. The sitting motions are easily accessible, reducing the danger of strain or injury while increasing flexibility and mobility.

2. Improved Flexibility: Regular chair yoga practice improves joint flexibility, which addresses common aging concerns including stiffness and limited range of motion. The carefully designed workouts emphasize moderate stretches that promote muscle and joint flexibility.

3. Increased Balance and Stability: The challenge includes exercises aimed at improving balance and stability, which are important for seniors. Participants can improve their balance by performing these motions, lowering their chance of falling and instilling more confidence in their regular activities.

4. Mind-Body Connection: Chair yoga promotes a strong mind-body connection via attentive movements and meditations. This blend of breath, movement, and mindfulness promotes mental clarity, stress reduction, and a general sense of wellbeing.

5. Joint Health: The sitting workouts in this challenge are intended to promote joint health. Seniors who engage in regulated and fluid motions can enhance joint lubrication, thus lowering the discomfort associated with illnesses such as arthritis.

6. Encourages relaxation and stress reduction: The challenge includes yoga nidra and visualization techniques to promote deep relaxation and stress reduction. Seniors can benefit from better sleep, less worry, and a stronger sense of inner serenity.

7. Tailored for Seniors: Recognizing seniors' special demands, the challenge includes workouts that take into account diminished mobility, joint sensitivity, and general comfort. The program is open to those with varied fitness levels and yoga experience.

8. Increases Energy Levels: The exercises are moderate, yet they are beneficial in increasing blood circulation and energy flow throughout the body. Seniors may experience a rise in vitality and energy levels, leading to a more active lifestyle.

9. Community Engagement: Participating in a 28-day challenge gives elders a feeling of camaraderie and common goals. This shared experience can promote motivation, solidarity, and a good attitude about wellness.

10. Empowerment and Independence: Chair yoga allows seniors to take charge of their health and well-being. Participants in an organized and realistic program may get a revitalized sense of independence and self-efficacy in controlling their physical and mental health.

CHAPTER 2
ESSENTIALS MATERIALS NEEDED

To start the 28 Days Chair Yoga for Seniors challenge, you'll need a few basic tools to guarantee a safe and pleasant practice. Here's a list of objects and why they're necessary:

1. Use a solid chair with a level seat and back support to maintain stability and balance during yoga poses.

- It serves as a solid basis for your practice and aids in the maintenance of appropriate posture throughout the exercises.

2. Wear loose, comfortable clothes for easy mobility and flexibility.

- Wearing comfortable clothing reduces constriction during stretches and enhances relaxation during meditation and breathing exercises.

3. Use a non-slip mat or yoga towel to keep your feet stable during sitting activities.

- It offers a pleasant surface for your feet, improving grip and stability during the practice.

4. Water Bottle: - Staying hydrated is crucial for any physical exercise, including chair yoga.

 - Keep a water bottle accessible to drink throughout the practice and replenish fluids lost from sweating and breathing.

5. Use a blanket or pillow for added support and comfort during sitting positions and relaxation techniques.

- Use it to elevate your knees or support your lower back, guaranteeing perfect alignment and decreasing joint strain.

6. Use a timer or clock to log your practice sessions.

- Setting a specific schedule helps you stay dedicated to your practice and ensures that you set aside adequate time for each workout and relaxation session.

7. Breath Awareness: - Yoga relies heavily on your breath.

- Throughout the exercises, breathe deeply and mindfully, inhaling and exhaling slowly and steadily.

- Conscious breathing improves relaxation, lowers tension, and strengthens the mind-body connection.

These tools are necessary for establishing a safe, pleasant, and productive chair yoga practice setting. They promote appropriate alignment, stability, and relaxation, allowing you to fully participate in the 28-day challenge and enjoy the advantages of chair yoga for elders.

SAFETY PRECAUTION

Before beginning the 28 Days Chair Yoga for Seniors challenge, prioritize safety to guarantee a happy and injury-free experience. Here are some critical safety measures to take before starting the challenge:

1. speak with Healthcare Provider: - Before starting a new fitness program, especially if you have pre-existing health concerns, speak with your healthcare provider to confirm chair yoga is appropriate for your requirements.

2. Pay attention to your body when exercising. If you encounter pain, discomfort, or dizziness, cease moving right away and seek medical attention if necessary.

3. Modify positions and exercises based on your fitness level and physical skills. Chair yoga is customizable, so choose movements that are comfortable and safe for you.

4. Use a Stable Chair: - Make sure your chair is stable, strong, and placed on a flat surface. Avoid chairs with wheels or instability, since they may represent a risk during specific motions.

5. Avoid overexertion. Chair yoga is intended to be gentle and restorative. Avoid overexertion and do not push yourself above your limitations. As you gain comfort and strength, gradually increase the intensity and length of your exercises.

6. Warm-Up and Cool Down: Start each session with a mild warm-up to prepare your body for action. Similarly, conclude with a soothing cool down to assist you return to a peaceful condition.

7. remain Hydrated: - Keep a water bottle nearby to remain hydrated throughout practice. Dehydration can lead to weariness and an increased risk of muscular cramping.

8. Use Props Safely: - When using props like pillows or blankets, make sure they are solid and non-slip. Place them appropriately to provide comfortable support for your body while maintaining safety.

9. Be attentive of your breathing. If you feel short of breath, revert to a comfortable breathing rhythm rather than straining it.

10. Practice in a Safe Environment: - Select a peaceful, well-lit area devoid of impediments to reduce the chance of stumbling or bumping against things while practice.

By taking these steps, you may create a safe and supportive setting for your chair yoga practice. Always prioritize your well-being, and if you have any issues or questions regarding specific exercises, consult with a trained teacher or healthcare expert.

CHAPTER 3
Day 1: Neck And Shoulder Mobility

INTRODUCTION: Gentle neck and shoulder exercises are essential for maintaining flexibility and reducing strain. These motions can help you improve your posture, reduce stiffness, and relieve pain. Before you begin, choose a peaceful and comfortable area, sit erect in your chair, and take a few deep breaths.

1. NECK TILTS (5 MINS):

- Begin by sitting tall, with your shoulders relaxed.

- Slowly tilt your head to onc side, bringing your ear near your shoulder.

- Hold the stretch for a few seconds, feeling the soft stretch on the other side of your neck.

- Repeat on the opposite side.

- Repeat 8-10 times on each side, moving at a moderate speed.

- Take it slowly and don't push any movements. Feel the stretch without pain.

2. SHOULDER ROLLS (5 MINS):

- Relax your arms at your sides.

- Lift your shoulders gently towards your ears and roll them back in a circular manner.

- Continue the circular motion for around ten times.

- Repeat 10 times in the other direction, rolling your shoulders forward.

- Concentrate on smooth and controlled motions, breathing normally throughout.

3. NECK ROTATIONS (5 MINS):

- Begin with your head in a neutral position.

- Slowly move your head to one side, bringing your chin to your shoulder.

- Hold the posture for a few seconds while feeling the strain in your neck.

- Return to the middle, then repeat on the opposite side.

- Do 8-10 revolutions on each side, moving at a moderate speed.

- Avoid making quick moves and listen to your body.

CONCLUSION: Completing these simple neck and shoulder movements is a terrific way to begin your chair yoga adventure. The emphasis on moderate and controlled movements improves mobility while minimizing muscular tension. Remember to relax and enjoy the revitalizing benefits. Take these exercises at your own pace, and if anything seems difficult, make changes or skip the action. Consistency is crucial, and you'll most likely feel more flexibility and less stiffness in your neck and shoulders with time.

INTRODUCTION: Seated side stretches are great for increasing spinal flexibility and torso range of motion. These exercises also work the muscles on your sides, which improves general mobility and comfort. Sit comfortably in your chair, feet flat on the floor, and take a minute to focus yourself before starting.

1. SIDE BEND STRETCH (5 MINS):

- Sit up straight, feet level on the floor.

- Inhale and raise your arms upwards, clasping your hands.

- Gently lean to one side, stretching the opposing side of your torso.

- Hold the stretch for 15-20 seconds while inhaling deeply.

- Return to the middle, then repeat on the opposite side.

- Do 5-8 stretches on each side at a calm and controlled rate.

2. SEATED TWISTS (5 MINS):

- Sit comfortably, feet hip-width apart.

- Inhale, stretching your spine, then exhale, twisting your torso to one side.

- For further support, place one hand on the outside of the opposing knee.

- Hold the twist for 15-20 seconds, experiencing a mild rotation in your spine.

- Return to the middle, then repeat on the opposite side.

- Make 5-8 twists on each side, moving easily and without tension.

3. SEATED SIDE STRETCH WITH ARM REACH (5 MINS):

- Sit with your back straight and your feet flat on the ground.

- Raise one arm overhead, reaching to the opposing side.

- Feel the stretch along your side while avoiding leaning forward.

- Hold the stretch for 15-20 seconds while inhaling deeply.

- Return to the middle, then repeat on the opposite side.

- Stretch 5-8 times on each side, keeping the action mild and controlled.

CONCLUSION: Seated side stretches make the body more flexible and supple. These workouts reduce spinal strain and improve your general well-being. As with any new activity, begin softly and gradually build in intensity. Consistency is essential to reaping the full advantages. Remember to breathe deeply throughout each stretch, and if you experience any pain, ease off or talk with your healthcare professional. These stretches are intended to be pleasurable and accessible, ensuring a good experience as you continue your chair yoga practice.

INTRODUCTION: Wrist and hand workouts are vital for preserving dexterity, decreasing stiffness, and improving circulation. These mild movements might be particularly good for folks who spend lengthy hours utilizing their hands. Begin in a comfortable sitting position, with your back supported and your feet firmly on the floor.

1. WRIST CIRCLES (5 MINS):

- Extend your arms in front of you, palms down.

- Start forming gentle circles with your wrists, going clockwise.

- After ten rounds, switch to counterclockwise rotation.

- Concentrate on the sensations in your wrists and forearm.

- Complete three sets of ten spins in each direction.

- If you experience any pain, limit your range of motion.

2. FINGER TAPS AND EXTENSIONS (5 MINS):

- Place your hands on your thighs, palms facing downward.

- Lift one finger at a time, beginning with your thumbs and progressing to your pinky.

- After elevating each finger, stretch it as far outward as possible.

- Repeat the steps, tapping and stretching each finger separately.

- Continue for three sets at a steady, methodical pace.

- This workout helps your fingers become more flexible and stronger.

3. HAND SQUEEZES WITH RESISTANCE (5 MINS):

- Hold a soft ball or stress ball in one hand.

- Squeeze the ball lightly and hold it for a few seconds.

- Release the pressure and stretch your fingers widely.

- Repeat the pattern 10 times, then switch to the other hand.

- Concentrate on the sensation of muscles functioning in your hands and fingers.

- This exercise improves grip strength and flexibility.

CONCLUSION: Taking care of your hands and wrists is essential for preserving freedom and comfort in everyday tasks. The exercises offered are intended to be moderate but useful in increasing flexibility and strength. As with any new practice, begin carefully and listen to your body. If you encounter pain or discomfort, reduce the intensity or speak with your doctor. Incorporating these exercises into your everyday routine can help to improve hand and wrist function over time. Enjoy the procedure and the feeling of enhanced mobility in your hands.

Day 4: Ankle Rolls and Toe Taps

INTRODUCTION: Ankle and toe exercises help to improve circulation, reduce edema, and preserve flexibility in the lower extremities. These motions are very useful for people who spend a lot of time sitting. Begin these exercises in a comfortable sitting position, feet flat on the floor.

1. ANKLE ROLLS (5 MINS):

- Lift one foot slightly off the floor while keeping the heel grounded.

- Rotate your ankle in a circular manner, starting clockwise.\

- After 10 revolutions, change to counterclockwise rotations.

- Repeat the process with the opposite foot.

- Do three sets of ten rotations in each direction for each ankle.

- Concentrate on the moderate stretch and range of motion in your ankles.

2. TOE TAPS (5 MINS):

- Raise your toes off the floor while keeping your heels grounded.

- Tap your toes on the floor for ten times.

- After tapping, pull your toes up and spread them out.

- Repeat the procedure three times, alternating between tapping and toe spreading.

- This exercise improves flexibility in the toes and tops of your feet

- Perform the exercise at a comfortable rate for you.

3. SEATED LEG EXTENSIONS (5 MINS):

- Sit comfortably, back straight and feet flat on the floor.

- Extend one leg forward and lift it slightly off the ground.

- Hold in the extended posture for a few seconds, experiencing a slight stretch in your hamstring.

- Return the leg to the floor and repeat with the other leg.

- Perform three sets of ten leg extensions for each leg.

- Practice smooth motions and avoid locking your knees.

CONCLUSION: Taking care of your ankles and toes is critical for preserving mobility and avoiding discomfort. These exercises are intended to be mild yet helpful in increasing flexibility and circulation in your lower limbs. As with any new exercise, begin gently and listen to your body. If you encounter pain or discomfort, reduce the intensity or speak with your doctor. Incorporating these ankle and toe exercises into your everyday routine can lead to increased comfort and flexibility over time. Enjoy the heightened sensation of mobility in your lower legs and feet.

Day 5: Deep Breathing Techniques

INTRODUCTION: Deep breathing techniques are an essential component of chair yoga, giving several benefits to both the body and mind. They relieve tension, enhance oxygen intake, and create a state of calm. These exercises may be done while sitting, making them accessible to everyone. Find a quiet, comfortable area, sit upright in your chair, and let's practice deep breathing together.

1. DIAPHRAGMATIC BREATHING (5 MINS):

- Sit comfortably, back straight and shoulders relaxed.

- Put one hand on your chest, the other on your abdomen.

- Take deep breaths through your nose, allowing your abdomen to expand.

- Feel your diaphragm descend as your lungs fill with air.

- Exhale gently and thoroughly through your lips, feeling your abdominal muscles tense.

- Repeat this technique for 5 minutes, concentrating on the rise and fall of your abdomen.

- This practice improves calm and increases oxygen flow.

2. EQUAL BREATHING (5 MINS):

- In a sitting position, inhale through your nose four times.

- Hold your breath for four counts.

- Exhale via your mouth four times.

- Pause momentarily before beginning the following cycle.

- Maintain an equal breathing pattern for 5 minutes.

- Keep a steady, comfortable pace throughout.

- This practice helps to regulate the breath and relax the nervous system.

3. 4-7-8 BREATHING (5 MINS):

- Sit comfortably with your back straight and your hands in your lap.

- Inhale gently through your nose for a count of four.

- Hold your breath for seven counts.

- Take a full, audible exhale through your mouth for eight counts.

- Continue the cycle for 5 minutes.

- Concentrate on the repetitive pattern and the relaxing impact on your body.

- This activity is proven to promote relaxation and reduce anxiety.

CONCLUSION: Deep breathing exercises are an effective strategy for enhancing both physical and mental health. The three strategies discussed today—Diaphragmatic Breathing, Equal Breathing, and 4-7-8 Breathing—are simple yet powerful ways to include mindful breathing into your everyday routine. Regularly practice these exercises to reduce stress, boost attention, and improve your sense of calm. As with any new discipline, begin with shorter sessions and progressively expand as you get more comfortable. As you progress through your chair yoga journey, enjoy the peaceful advantages of deep breathing.

Day 6: Introduction to Meditation

INTRODUCTION: Meditation is an excellent practice with multiple advantages for both the mind and body. It can help you relax, concentrate better, and feel more at ease. Today, we'll look at three meditation techniques ideal for beginners. Find a peaceful and comfortable area, sit erect in your chair, and let us begin our meditation trip.

1. GUIDED BODY SCAN MEDITATION (5 MINS):

- Sit comfortably with a straight back and hands on lap.

- If you feel comfortable, softly close your eyes.

- Begin by focusing your attention on your breathing, taking a few deep breaths to center yourself.

- Change your concentration to other regions of your body, beginning with your toes and up to the top of your head.

- As you concentrate on each body area, let go of any tension or discomfort you experience.

- Allow your breath to guide you through this procedure, paying attention to each location.

- Continue the body scan for 5 minutes, focusing on relaxation.

2. MINDFULNESS MEDITATION WITH BREATH (5 MINS):

- Sit comfortably and focus your attention on your breath.

- Inhale slowly through your nose while counting to four.

- Exhale slowly through your mouth while counting to four.

- Concentrate on the sensation of breath entering and exiting your body.

- If your thoughts begin to stray, softly redirect your attention back to your breath.

- Spend 5 minutes practicing this mindfulness meditation, allowing your breath to anchor your consciousness.

3. LOVING KINDNESS MEDITATION (5 MINS):

- Get comfortable, close your eyes, and take a few deep breaths.

- Start by channeling sentiments of love and kindness toward yourself.

- Say quietly or aloud sentences like "May I be happy, healthy, safe, and at ease."

- Extend these desires to others, beginning with someone you care about and subsequently expanding to others.

- Feel the warmth of these good thoughts emanating from your heart.

- Practice loving-kindness meditation for 5 minutes to cultivate compassion.

CONCLUSION: Meditation is a peaceful and transforming practice that may bring calm and insight into your life. Newcomers to meditation will benefit greatly from the guided body scan, awareness with breath, and loving-kindness meditation. Begin with short intervals and progressively expand as you gain comfort. Remember that meditation is a personal journey, with no right or wrong way to do it. Enjoy the moments of calm and presence as you learn about the advantages of meditation in your chair yoga regimen.

Day 7: Relaxation Pose

INTRODUCTION: Relaxation poses are a vital component of chair yoga, providing time for your body and mind to calm and recharge. Today, we'll look at three relaxation postures that help you feel peaceful and release stress. Find a peaceful and comfortable place, sit on your chair with your back supported, and let's dive into the realm of relaxation.

1. SEATED FORWARD BEND (5-MINS):

- sit comfortably with your back straight and feet flat on the floor.

- Inhale deeply to extend your spine.

- As you exhale, bend at the hips and softly lean forward, bringing your chest closer to your thighs.

- Let your arms hang loosely or rest on the floor in front of you.

- Hold the stretch for 5 minutes, inhaling deeply and letting go with each exhale.

- Feel a nice stretch around your spine and back of your legs.

2. CHAIR YOGA RECLINED POSE (5 MINS):

- Add a cushion or folded blanket to the back of your chair for support.

- Sit comfortably with your back against the support and let your head rest securely.

- Extend your legs and rest them on a footrest or the floor.

- Close your eyes and concentrate on your breathing, letting rid of any tension with each exhalation.

- Hold this reclining attitude for 5 minutes, allowing your body to fully rest.

- This position produces a feeling of comfort and relaxation throughout your body.

3. GUIDED VISUALIZATION (5 MINS):

- Sit comfortably, with your back straight and your hands resting on your lap.

- Gently close your eyes, or lessen your stare if it seems more comfortable.

- To center yourself, take a few deep breaths.

- Imagine a quiet location, such as a beach, a forest, or a meadow.

- Visualize the sights, sounds, and sensations of this peaceful setting.

- Spend 5 minutes immersing your senses in this vision, letting stress to melt away.

- When you're ready, slowly open your eyes while feeling rejuvenated and relaxed.

CONCLUSION: Chair yoga relies heavily on relaxation positions, which allow for profound rest and renewal. The sitting forward bend, chair yoga reclining posture, and guided visualization are all easy yet powerful techniques to relax. Incorporate these relaxation postures into your normal practice to give your body and mind the advantages of deep relaxation. As with any new discipline, begin with short sessions and progressively increase the duration as you feel more comfortable. Enjoy the relaxing and calming benefits of these postures, which will add a feeling of peace to your chair yoga journey.

Self-Assessment Journal - Week 1

DAY 1:

How did you feel during the neck and shoulder mobility exercises today? ---

----

Did you experience any discomfort or tension, and if so, how did you address it?--

----

Day 2:

Reflect on the seated side stretches. Were you able to feel a gentle stretch along your sides? ---

----

----

did you notice any changes in your flexibility? ----------------------

----

Day 3:

Share your experience with the wrist and hand exercises. Did you find them helpful in reducing stiffness? ----------------------------

----

were there any specific challenges you encountered?---------------

----

Day 4:

How did the ankle rolls and toe taps affect your lower extremities?

Did you notice any changes in circulation or a reduction in swelling? --

----

Day 5:

Reflect on the deep breathing techniques introduced today. Did you find it challenging to stay focused on your breath? ------------

----

----

did you notice any immediate effects on your stress levels?

Day 6: Explore your first day of meditation. How did you feel during and after the meditation session? -----------------------------

----

----

and were you able to maintain a sense of calm and focus? ---------

----

Day 7:

Consider your experience with the relaxation poses. Did you feel a sense of ease and relaxation? -------------------------------------

----

----

and did it contribute to a more peaceful state of mind?------------

----

CONCLUSION: As you reflect on the entire week's chair yoga practices, what benefits have you noticed so far? -------------------

----

Are there specific areas where you've observed improvement or areas that may need more attention in the coming weeks? ---------

----

Remember, this journal is a personal reflection tool, and there are no right or wrong answers. Use it as a way to track your progress, understand your body, and make adjustments to your chair yoga routine as needed.

CHAPTER 4

Day 8: Seated Twists

INTRODUCTION: Seated twists are great for increasing spinal flexibility and boosting digestion. These exercises are mild and can be done while seated, making them suitable for everyone. Today, we'll look at three types of sitting twists. Find a quiet, comfortable location, sit up straight in your chair, and let's improve our spinal mobility.

1. BASIC SEATED TWIST (5 MINS):

- Sit comfortably, back straight, feet flat on the floor.

- Inhale deeply to extend your spine.

- Exhale and twist your torso to one side, placing your hand on the back of the chair for support.

- Hold the twist for 15-20 seconds, experiencing a mild rotation in your spine.

- Inhale as you return to center, then exhale and twist to the opposite side.

- Repeat this exercise for 5 minutes, changing sides and emphasizing smooth, controlled motions.

- Notice the stretch throughout your spine and the mild contraction of your core.

2. SEATED TWIST WITH ARM REACH (5 MINS):

- Sit with your back straight and feet flat on the ground.

- Inhale and raise one arm overhead, reaching to the opposite side.

- Exhale while twisting your torso to the side and bringing the elevated arm across your body.

- Hold the twist for 15-20 seconds, feeling the stretch on your side and spine.

- Inhale back into the center, then repeat on the opposite side.

- Continue this routine for 5 minutes at a slow, controlled pace.

- This variant provides an extra stretch for your side muscles.

3. SEATED CHAIR TWIST FLOW (5 MINS):

- Sit comfortably, with your hands on the armrests or seat of the chair.

- Inhale and extend your spine while activating your core.

- Exhale as you rotate your torso to one side, placing your opposing hand on the back of the chair.

- Inhale back into the center, then exhale and twist to the opposite side.

- Continue this flow for 5 minutes, moving with your breath.

- Concentrate on the steady, rhythmic movement and feel the energy flow through your spine.

- This flowing variant adds dynamic movement to the sitting twist.

CONCLUSION: Seated twists are an excellent approach to improve spine flexibility and maintain a healthy range of motion. The basic seated twist, seated twist with arm reach, and sitting chair twist flow offer modifications to fit a variety of tastes. Practice these exercises on a daily basis to improve your spine's mobility. As with any new exercise, begin with short sessions and progressively expand as you feel more comfortable. Enjoy the fluidity and subtle stretch that these sitting twists provide to your chair yoga practice.

Day 9: Abdominal Contractions

INTRODUCTION: Abdominal contractions help to develop the core muscles, which are responsible for supporting your spine and maintaining balance. These exercises are intended to be gentle but effective, improving balance and overall well-being. Find a comfortable seated posture in your chair, with your back well-supported, and let's start working on our core strength.

1. SEATED MARCHING (5 MINS):

- Sit comfortably, back straight, feet flat on the floor.

- Inhale deeply while activating your core muscles.

- Exhale while lifting one leg to your chest, as if you were marching in place.

- Lower the elevated leg to the floor and repeat on the opposite side.

- Repeat this marching action for 5 minutes, keeping a consistent tempo.

- As you elevate your knees, pay attention to how your abdominal muscles engage.

- This workout strengthens your core and improves circulation in the legs.

2. PELVIC TILTS (5 MINS):

- Sit comfortably, feet hip-width apart, hands resting on your thighs.

- Inhale deeply to extend your spine.

- Exhale by tilting your pelvis forward and rounding your lower back.

- Inhale to return to a neutral position, then exhale and tilt your pelvis backward, arching your lower back.

- Continue rocking for 5 minutes, concentrating on the movement of your pelvis.

- Pelvic tilts activate your core and help to improve posture.

3. SEATED ABDOMINAL SQUEEZE (5 MINS):

- Sit comfortably, with your back straight and your hands resting on your lap.

- Inhale deeply, widening your chest.

- Exhale while engaging your abdominal muscles and pulling them slightly towards your spine.

- Hold the contraction for a few seconds before inhaling and exhaling.

- Repeat the abdominal squeeze for 5 minutes, concentrating on the controlled contraction and release.

- This exercise works the deep muscles of your core, increasing strength and stability.

CONCLUSION: Abdominal contractions are an excellent supplement to any chair yoga exercise, giving important core strength benefits. Seated marching, pelvic tilts, and seated abdominal squeezes are all versions that target distinct elements of your core muscles. Practice these exercises on a regular basis to enhance spinal stability and support. As with any new exercise, begin with short sessions and progressively expand as you feel more comfortable. Enjoy the strengthening effects of these abdominal contractions as you continue your chair yoga adventure.

INTRODUCTION: Pelvic tilts and raises are excellent exercises for developing core strength, flexibility, and stability. These exercises work the muscles in your lower back, hips, and abdomen, promoting total spinal health. Find a comfortable sitting position in your chair, with sufficient back support, and then focus on these helpful activities.

1. SEATED PELVIC TILTS (5 MINS):

- Sit comfortably, feet flat on the floor and hands resting on your thighs.

- Inhale deeply, stretching your spine and activating your core.

- Exhale by tilting your pelvis forward and arching your lower back.

- Inhale to return to the neutral posture.

- Exhale by tilting your pelvis backward and rounding your lower back.

- Continue rocking for 5 minutes, matching your breathing with the movement.

- Pelvic tilts promote lower-back flexibility and core awareness.

2. SEATED PELVIC LIFTS (5 MINS):

- Sit comfortably, with your hands on the chair's armrests or seat for support.

- Inhale deeply while activating your core muscles.

- Exhale as you lift your pelvis off the chair and move your weight to your feet.

- Inhale and drop your pelvis back down.

- Repeat the lifting action for 5 minutes at a moderate pace.

- Concentrate on improving your core strength and pelvic control.

- Pelvic lifts work the muscles in your lower abdomen and improve overall core strength.

3. SEATED FIGURE-EIGHT PELVIC MOVEMENTS (5 MINS):

- Sit comfortably, back straight, feet flat on the floor.

- Take a deep inhale and engage your core.

- Exhale and move your hips in a circular manner to form a figure-eight pattern.

- Continue this flowing movement for 5 minutes, harmonizing your breathing with the figure-eight motion.

- Concentrate on the delicate engagement of your core and the smoothness of pelvic motions.

- This exercise improves hip mobility and provides relaxation in the lower back.

CONCLUSION: Pelvic tilts and lifts provide several advantages for your core and lower back health. The sitting pelvic tilts, lifts, and figure-eight pelvic motions all work various muscle areas. Practice these exercises on a regular basis to increase core strength, flexibility, and stability. As with any new exercise, begin with short sessions and progressively expand as you feel more comfortable. Enjoy the flexibility and strength-building benefits of these pelvic movements as you continue your chair yoga adventure.

Day 11: Leg Strengthening Exercises

INTRODUCTION: Leg strengthening workouts are essential for preserving mobility, stability, and general leg health. These mild yet efficient motions target the muscles in your thighs, hips, and lower legs. Find a comfortable sitting position in your chair, with sufficient back support, and then perform these helpful leg exercises.

1. SEATED LEG EXTENSIONS (5 MINS):

- Sit comfortably, back straight, feet flat on the floor.

- Inhale deeply while activating your core muscles.

- Exhale as you straighten one leg in front of you, elevating it slightly off the ground.

- Inhale and drop the leg back down.

- Repeat the extension with your other leg.

- Continue alternating leg extensions for 5 minutes, moving at a moderate speed.

- Concentrate on activating your thigh muscles and moving your legs with control.

- Seated leg extensions serve to strengthen the thighs and increase leg endurance.

2. SEATED KNEE LIFTS (5 MINS):

- Sit comfortably, back upright and hands resting on the chair's armrests or seat.

- Take a deep inhale and engage your core.

- Exhale as you raise one leg to your chest, as high as you feel comfortable.

- Inhale and drop the knee back down.

- Repeat the knee lift with your second leg.

- Continue alternating knee lifts for 5 minutes at a moderate pace.

- Work on strengthening your hip flexors and controlling your knee movement.

- Seated knee lifts work the muscles in your hips and help to increase leg strength.

3. SEATED HEEL RAISES (5 MINS):

- Sit comfortably, back straight, feet flat on the floor.

- Take a deep inhale and engage your core.

- Exhale as you raise both heels off the floor, landing on the balls of your feet.

- Inhale to bring the heels back down.

  Repeat the heel lift for 5 minutes, moving at a moderate speed.

- Concentrate on contracting your calf muscles and moving your feet with control.

- Seated heel rises serve to strengthen the calves and improve ankle stability.

CONCLUSION: Leg strengthening exercises are vital for maintaining the mobility and strength of your lower legs. The seated leg extensions, knee lifts, and heel raises are versions that work distinct muscle groups. Practice these exercises on a daily basis to enhance leg strength, stability, and endurance. As with any new exercise, begin with short sessions and progressively expand as you feel more comfortable. Enjoy the leg strengthening benefits of these exercises as you continue your chair yoga adventure.

Day 12: Balance and Stability Exercises

INTRODUCTION: Balance and stability exercises are essential for maintaining control, avoiding falls, and improving general health. These motions are intended to be moderate and may be performed while seated in a chair, with an emphasis on activating the muscles that contribute to stability. Find a comfortable sitting posture with enough back support, and then try some healthy balancing exercises.

1. SEATED MARCHING WITH BALANCE (5 MINS):

- Sit comfortably, back straight, feet flat on the floor.

- Inhale deeply while activating your core muscles.

- Exhale and lift one leg to your chest, holding it for a few seconds.

- Inhale to bring the foot back to the ground.

- Repeat the marching motion with your other leg.

- Continue alternating sitting marching with balancing for 5 minutes, moving at a moderate speed.

- Maintain stability as you elevate each knee.

- Seated marching with balance improves core strength and stability.

2. SEATED LEG CROSSES (5 MIN):

- Sit comfortably, back straight, feet flat on the floor.

- Inhale deeply while activating your core muscles.

- Exhale while lifting one foot slightly off the ground and crossing it over the opposing knee.

- Hold the crossing posture for a few seconds while feeling the stretch in your hip.

- Inhale to bring the foot back to the ground.

- Repeat the leg cross with your other leg.

- Repeat the alternating sitting leg crosses for 5 minutes, moving at a moderate speed.

- Maintain stability and balance when crossing the legs.

- Seated leg crosses work the muscles involved for hip stability.

3. SEATED HEEL-TO-TOE TAP (5 MIN):

- Sit comfortably, back straight, feet flat on the floor.

- Inhale deeply while activating your core muscles.

- Exhale as you lift one foot slightly off the floor, tapping the heel on the toe of the opposing foot.

- Inhale to bring the foot back to the ground.

- Repeat the heel-to-toe tap with the second foot.

- Repeat the alternate sitting heel-to-toe tap for 5 minutes, moving at a moderate speed.

- Concentrate on maintaining stability and control throughout the tapping action.

- Seated heel-to-toe taps improve coordination and stability.

CONCLUSION: Balance and stability exercises are critical for maintaining control and avoiding falls. The sitting marching with balance, leg crosses, and heel-to-toe tap exercises are versions that work distinct muscle areas associated with stability. To enhance your balance and stability, do these exercises on a daily basis. As with any new exercise, begin with short sessions and progressively expand as you feel more comfortable. As you progress through your chair yoga practice, enjoy the sensation of control and stability that these movements provide.

Day 13: Gentle Neck and Shoulder Releases

INTRODUCTION: Gentle neck and shoulder exercises can assist to reduce stress, increase flexibility, and promote relaxation. These exercises are intended to be relaxing and easy to practice while sitting in a chair. Find a comfortable sitting position with enough back support, and then explore these healthy neck and shoulder releases.

1. NECK TILTS AND TURNS (5 MINS):

- Sit comfortably, back straight, shoulders relaxed.

- Inhale deeply, then as you exhale, gradually tilt your head to one side, bringing your ear near your shoulder.

- Hold the stretch for a few seconds until you feel a mild release on the side of your neck.

- Inhale to bring your head back to an upright posture.

- Exhale and tilt your head to the opposite side.

- Continue this mild tilting action for 5 minutes, at a comfortable pace.

- Next, slowly rotate your head to the left and right.

- This exercise helps to relieve stress in the neck and enhances range of motion.

2. SHOULDER ROLLS (5 MINS):

- Sit comfortably, with your back straight and your hands resting on your lap.

- Take a deep inhale, and as you exhale, raise your shoulders towards your ears.

- Inhale, then rotate your shoulders backward in a circular manner.

- As you complete the circle, exhale and bring your shoulders down.

- Repeat the shoulder rolling action for 5 minutes, concentrating on the slow release of tension.

- After several minutes, reverse the direction of the shoulder rolls.

- This exercise helps to alleviate tension in the shoulder muscles.

3. SEATED NECK STRETCHES (5 MINS):

- Sit comfortably, with your back straight and your hands resting on your lap.

- Inhale deeply, then as you exhale, tilt your head forward and bring your chin to your chest.

- Hold the stretch for a few seconds to feel a slight elongation down the back of your neck.

- Inhale to bring your head back to an upright posture.

- Exhale and tilt your head back, staring at the ceiling.

- Continue gently stretching for 5 minutes at a comfortable pace.

- This exercise helps to relieve stress in the neck and upper back.

CONCLUSION: Gentle neck and shoulder releases are essential for preserving comfort and flexibility. Neck tilts and rotations, shoulder rolls, and sitting neck stretches all offer variants that target specific regions of stress. Practice these exercises on a regular basis to enhance relaxation and eliminate stiffness in your neck and shoulders. As with any new exercise, begin with short sessions and progressively expand as you feel more comfortable. Enjoy the calming benefits of these mild releases as you continue your chair yoga journey.

INTRODUCTION: Mindful breathing and meditation are effective activities that promote calm, attention, and general well-being. These exercises may be completed while sitting on a chair, making them accessible to everyone. Find a comfortable sitting posture with enough back support, and let's begin this journey of inner calm.

1. MINDFUL BREATH AWARENESS (5 MINS):

- Sit comfortably, with your back straight and your hands resting on your lap.

- If you feel comfortable, softly close your eyes.

- To center yourself, take a few deep breaths.

- Bring your attention to your breath, observing each inhalation and exhale.

- As you inhale, remind yourself, **"I am aware that I am breathing in."**

- As you exhale, remind yourself, **"I am aware that I am breathing out."**

- Continue this focused breath awareness for 5 minutes, concentrating on the feeling of your breathing.

- If your mind wanders, softly return your concentration to your breathing.

- This activity encourages a sense of presence and calm.

2. GUIDED LOVING-KINDNESS MEDITATION (5 MINS):

- Sit comfortably with your back straight and hands on your lap.

- Gently close your eyes, or lessen your stare if it seems more comfortable.

- To center yourself, take a few deep breaths.

- Start by channeling sentiments of love and kindness toward yourself.

- Say quietly or aloud sentences **like "May I be happy, healthy, safe, and at ease."**

- Extend these desires to others, beginning with someone you care about and subsequently expanding to others.

- Feel the warmth of these good thoughts emanating from your heart.

- Practice loving-kindness meditation for 5 minutes to cultivate compassion.

- This meditation encourages sentiments of love and connection.

3. BODY SCAN MEDITATION (5 MINS):

- Sit comfortably, with your back straight and your hands resting on your lap.

- If you feel comfortable, softly close your eyes.

- To center yourself, take a few deep breaths.

- Start bringing your awareness to different regions of your body, beginning with your toes and up to the top of your head.

- As you concentrate on each body area, let go of whatever tension or discomfort you experience.

- Allow your breath to lead you through this procedure, paying attention to each location.

- Continue the body scan for 5 minutes, focusing on relaxation.

- This meditation encourages the connection between the mind and the body.

CONCLUSION: Mindful breathing and meditation are extremely useful skills for promoting calm and well-being. Mindful breath awareness, guided loving-kindness meditation, and body scan meditation all allow opportunities to study distinct facets of mindfulness. Regularly practice these exercises to reduce stress, boost attention, and improve your sense of calm. As with any new exercise, begin with short sessions and progressively expand as you feel more comfortable. As you go through your chair yoga journey, enjoy the calm and awareness that these techniques provide.

DAY 8:

How did the seated twists feel today? ---------------------------------

----

Did you notice any improvements in your spinal flexibility or overall comfort during the exercises? ----------------------------

----

DAY 9:

Reflect on the abdominal contraction exercises. Were you able to engage your core effectively? -----------------------------------

----

Did you experience any changes in how you perceive your core strength? --

----

DAY 10:

Share your experience with the pelvic tilts and lifts. Did you feel more aware of your pelvic movement? ----------------------------------

----

Did these exercises contribute to a sense of stability in your core? --

----

Day 11:

How did the leg strengthening exercises impact your lower

extremities? --

Did you notice any changes in leg strength or stability during the

seated leg extensions, knee lifts, and heel raises? -------------------

----

DAY 12:

Reflect on the balance and stability Exercises. Did you find the

seated marching with balance, leg crosses, and heel-to-toe tap

beneficial for enhancing your sense of stability? -------------------

----

DAY 13:

How did the gentle neck and shoulder releases feel today? --------

----

Did you experience a reduction in tension and increased comfort

in your neck and shoulder muscles? -----------------------------------

----

DAY 14:

Share your experience with the mindful breathing and meditation

practices. Did you notice any changes in your mental state, focus,

or overall sense of well-being during these mindfulness exercises?

CONCLUSION: As you reflect on the entire week's chair yoga practices, what improvements or changes have you observed in your physical comfort, mental well-being, or overall experience? -

----

Are there specific exercises or aspects of the routine that you find particularly beneficial or challenging and why? ---------------------

----

WE ARE HALF WAY THROUGH THIS CHALLENGE

STAY FOCUSED AND MOTIVATED

1. Progress Takes Time: readers should understand that progress does not occur instantly. It is common to encounter hurdles and failures along the route. be patient and to recognize even minor accomplishments.

2. Emphasize the multiple health advantages of chair yoga, including increased flexibility, less stress, higher mindfulness, better posture, and improved general well-being. Emphasize that persistence is essential for reaping these advantages.

3. Listen to Your Body: readers should listen to their bodies and make changes as necessary. Chair yoga is suitable to a variety of fitness levels and physical capabilities.

CHAPTER 5
Day 15: Seated Cardio Workout

INTRODUCTION: Seated cardio activities improve circulation, energy levels, and general cardiovascular health. These exercises are intended to be moderate, effective, and manageable while sitting in a chair. Find a comfortable sitting posture with sufficient back support, and let's begin our journey to enhance cardiovascular fitness.

1. SEATED MARCHING WITH ARM SWINGS (5-MINS):

- Sit comfortably, back straight, feet flat on the floor.

- Inhale deeply while activating your core muscles.

- Exhale as you bring one leg to your chest and swing the opposing arm forward.

- Inhale to bring the foot back down.

- Repeat the marching motion with the second leg, swinging the other arm.

- Continue alternating sitting marching with arm swings for 5 minutes, moving at a moderate speed.

- Concentrate on engaging your core and using your arms with control.

- This workout stimulates cardiovascular activity and boosts blood flow.

2. SEATED JUMPING JACKS (5-MINS):

- Sit comfortably, back straight, feet flat on the floor.

- Take a deep inhale and engage your core.

- Exhale while lifting both arms above and extending your legs to the sides.

- Inhale and drop your arms, then bring your legs back together.

- Repeat the motion for 5 minutes at a moderate speed.

- Concentrate on the rhythmic movement and involvement of your upper and lower bodies.

- Seated jumping jacks increase your heart rate and improve cardiovascular fitness.

3. SEATED HIGH KNEE TAPS (5 MINS):

- Sit comfortably, back straight and hands resting on your thighs.

- Take a deep inhale and engage your core.

- Exhale and lift one knee to your chest, tapping it with the opposing hand.

- Inhale to bring the foot back down.

- Repeat the high knee tap with your second leg.

- Repeat the alternating high knee tapping action for 5 minutes at a steady pace.

- Concentrate on increasing your heart rate and moving your legs with control.

- Seated high knee taps give a good cardiovascular exercise while sitting.

CONCLUSION: Seated cardio workouts are a great approach to improve cardiovascular health and boost energy levels. Sitting marching with arm swings, jumping jacks, and high knee taps offer variants that work different muscular areas. Practice these exercises on a daily basis to improve your circulation, cardiovascular fitness, and general health. As with any new exercise, begin with short sessions and progressively expand as you feel more comfortable. Enjoy the heart-healthy advantages of these sitting cardio exercises as you continue your chair yoga adventure.

Day 16: Heel and Toe Taps

INTRODUCTION: Heel and toe taps are easy workouts that increase ankle flexibility, circulation, and lower leg strength. These routines are simple to complete while sitting, making them appropriate for people of all fitness levels. Find a comfortable sitting posture with enough back support, and let's look at the advantages of heel and toe tapping.

1. SEATED HEEL TAPS (5 MINS):

- Sit comfortably, back straight, feet flat on the floor.

- Take a deep inhale and engage your core.

- Exhale as you lift your heels off the floor and bring them to your buttocks.

- Inhale and drop your heels back down.

- Repeat the heel tapping action for 5 minutes at a steady pace.

- Concentrate on the controlled movement of your heels and the contraction of your calf muscles.

- Seated heel taps enhance ankle flexibility and strengthen your calves.

2. SEATED TOE TAPS (5 MINS):

- Sit comfortably, back straight, feet flat on the floor.

- Take a deep inhale and engage your core.

- Exhale as you lift the balls of your feet off the ground, tapping your toes in place.

- Inhale to bring your toes back down.

- Repeat the toe tapping action for 5 minutes at a steady pace.

- Concentrate on controlling the movement of your toes and using your shin muscles.

- Seated toe taps enhance ankle flexibility and strengthen the muscles in your shin.

3. SEATED HEEL-TO-TOE TAPS (5 MINS):

- Sit comfortably, back straight, feet flat on the floor.

- Take a deep inhale and engage your core.

- Exhale while lifting your heels off the ground, then tap the balls of your feet.

- Inhale and drop your feet back to the beginning position.

- Repeat the heel-to-toe tapping action for 5 minutes, moving at a comfortable speed.

- Concentrate on the synchronized movement of your heels and toes.

- Seated heel-to-toe taps offer a complete exercise for ankle flexibility and lower leg strength.

CONCLUSION: Heel and toe taps are great exercises for increasing ankle flexibility and strengthening the muscles in your lower legs. The sitting heel taps, toe taps, and heel-to-toe taps all work distinct parts of your lower leg muscles. Practice these exercises on a daily basis to increase circulation, flexibility, and strength in your ankles and lower legs. As with any new exercise, begin with short sessions and progressively expand as you feel more comfortable. Enjoy the advantages of these heel and toe taps as you continue your chair yoga practice.

INTRODUCTION: Side leg raises are effective workouts for strengthening the muscles in your hips and thighs. These activities help to develop hip stability, balance, and total lower body strength. Find a comfortable sitting position with enough back support, and then explore the advantages of side leg lifts.

1. SEATED SIDE LEG RAISES (5 MINS):

- Sit comfortably, with your back straight and your hands resting on your lap.

- Inhale deeply while activating your core muscles.

- Exhale and lift one leg to the side, maintaining it straight.

- Inhale and drop the leg back down.

- Repeat the side leg lift with your second leg.

- Repeat this alternating side leg lifting action for 5 minutes at a moderate speed.

- Concentrate on activating your outer hip muscles and moving your legs with control.

- Seated side leg raises develop the muscles in your hips and thighs, which improves stability.

2. SEATED CROSS LEG LIFTS (5 MINS):

- Sit comfortably, with your back straight and your hands resting on your lap.

- Take a deep inhale and engage your core.

- Exhale as you raise one leg and cross it over the other while maintaining both legs straight.

- Inhale and drop the leg back down.

- Repeat the cross-leg raise with your other leg.

- Repeat this alternating cross leg lifting action for 5 minutes, moving at a moderate speed.

- Concentrate on engaging your inner and outer thigh muscles, as well as moving your legs with control.

- Seated cross leg lifts give a thorough workout for your thighs.

3. SEATED LEG CIRCLES (5 MINS):

- Sit comfortably, with your back straight and your hands resting on your lap.

- Take a deep inhale and engage your core.

- Exhale while lifting one leg and drawing little circles in the air.

- Inhale to reverse the orientation of the circle.

- Repeat the leg circles with your second leg.

- Continue this alternating leg circular motion for 5 minutes at a moderate speed.

- Concentrate on the controlled movement of your legs and the contraction of your hip muscles.

- Seated leg circles increase hip flexibility and strengthen the muscles surrounding the hip joint.

CONCLUSION: Side leg raises are a terrific workout for improving hip stability and strengthening your thighs. The sitting side leg rises, cross leg lifts, and leg circles are all versions that target distinct muscular areas in your lower body. Regular practice of these exercises will result in better hip strength, stability, and general lower body function. As with any new exercise, begin with short sessions and progressively expand as you feel more comfortable. Enjoy the advantages of these side leg lifts as you continue your chair yoga adventure.

Day 18: Chair Yoga Warrior Pose

INTRODUCTION: The Chair Yoga Warrior Pose is a modified variation of the standard Warrior Pose that can be practiced sitting. This stance is ideal for increasing strength, stability, and attention. Find a comfortable sitting posture with enough back support, and then experience the advantages of the Chair Yoga Warrior Pose.

1. FOR SEATED WARRIOR I (5 MINS):

- sit comfortably with your back straight and feet flat on the floor.

- Take a deep inhale and engage your core.

- Exhale and stretch one leg forward, keeping the foot on the ground and the knee slightly bent.

- Inhale as you raise both arms aloft and bring your palms together.

- Exhale, then maintain the posture for a few seconds, feeling the stretch in your arms and extended leg.

- Inhale to drop your arms and return the foot to its initial position.

- Repeat Seated Warrior I on the opposite side.

- Repeat this alternating Seated Warrior I motion for 5 minutes at a moderate pace.

- Focus on your core's strength and stability, as well as the stretch in your arms and legs.

2. SEATED WARRIOR II (5-MINS):

- Sit comfortably, back straight, feet flat on the floor.

- Take a deep inhale and engage your core.

- Exhale while extending one leg to the side, with the foot on the floor and the knee slightly bent.

- Inhale as you spread your arms wide, parallel to the floor, palms down.

- Exhale, then maintain the posture for a few seconds, feeling the stretch in your arms and extended leg.

- Inhale to bring your arms back to the center and your foot to the beginning position.

- Repeat Seated Warrior II on the opposite side.

- Continue this alternating Seated Warrior II motion for 5 minutes at a moderate pace.

- Concentrate on the strength and stability of your core, the stretch in your arms, and the extended leg.

3. SEATED WARRIOR III (5-MINS):

- Sit comfortably, back straight, feet flat on the floor.

- Take a deep inhale and engage your core.

- Exhale as you lean forward and extend one leg straight behind you, parallel to the ground.

- Inhale while reaching your arms forward, forming a straight line from your fingers to your extended foot.

- Exhale and hold the stance for a few seconds, feeling the core engage and the leg stretch.

- Inhale to return to your starting position.

- Repeat Seated Warrior III on the opposite side.

- Repeat this alternating Seated Warrior III motion for 5 minutes at a moderate pace.

- Concentrate on the strength and stability of your core, the stretch in your arms, and the extended leg.

CONCLUSION: The Chair Yoga Warrior Pose series is a powerful collection of exercises that improve strength, stability, and attention. The Seated Warrior I, II, and III are versions that target distinct muscle areas. Practice these exercises on a regular basis to enhance your strength, stability, and sensation of empowerment. As with any new exercise, begin with short sessions and progressively expand as you feel more comfortable. Enjoy the advantages of the Chair Yoga Warrior Pose series as you continue your chair yoga adventure

INTRODUCTION: The Tree Pose with Support is a moderate variation on the standard Tree Pose that is performed while seated and using a chair for balance. This position improves stability, leg strength, and attention. Find a comfortable sitting posture with enough back support, and then discover the advantages of the Tree Pose with Support.

1. SEATED TREE POSE (5 MINS):

- Sit comfortably, back straight, feet flat on the floor.

- Take a deep inhale and engage your core.

- Exhale as you lift one foot off the ground, resting the sole against the inner thigh or calf of the opposing leg.

- If necessary, place your hands on the chair's back to provide support.

- Inhale to stretch your spine; exhale to relax into the position.

- Hold the Seated Tree Pose for a few seconds, concentrating on your breath and the connection between your foot and inner thigh/calf.

- Inhale to drop the foot back to the floor, then repeat on the opposite side.

- Hold this alternate seated tree pose for 5 minutes at a steady pace.

- Concentrate on the stability offered by the chair and the stretch in your legs.

2. SUPPORTED LEG EXTENSION (5 MINS):

- Sit comfortably, back straight, feet flat on the floor.

- Take a deep inhale and engage your core.

- Exhale while you raise one leg forward, parallel to the ground.

- For support, hold the back of the chair, with a small bend in the knee if necessary.

- Inhale to stretch your spine, then exhale and hold the Supported Leg Extension for a few seconds.

- Inhale to bring the foot back to the ground.

- Repeat the supported leg extension on the opposite side.

- Repeat the alternate Supported Leg Extension for 5 minutes, moving at a moderate speed.

- Concentrate on the support offered by the chair and the engagement of your extended leg.

3. SEATED ANKLE-TO-KNEE POSE (5 MINS):

- Sit comfortably, back straight, feet flat on the floor.

- Take a deep inhale and engage your core.

- Exhale as you lift one foot off the floor and place the ankle on the opposing knee.

- Use the chair for support, with your hands on the back.

- Inhale to stretch your spine, then exhale to go into the Seated Ankle-to-Knee Pose.

- Hold the stance for a few seconds, focusing on the stretch in the hip of the crossed leg.

- Inhale to drop the foot back to the floor, then repeat on the opposite side.

- Hold this alternating seated ankle-to-knee pose for 5 minutes at a steady pace.

- Pay attention to the chair's support and the slight stretch in your hips.

CONCLUSION: The Tree Pose with Support series is an excellent combination of exercises for increasing stability, leg strength, and attention. The Seated Tree Pose, Supported Leg Extension, and Seated Ankle-to-Knee Pose are all versions that target distinct muscle groups. Practice these exercises on a daily basis to enhance your balance, strength, and feeling of grounding.

Day 20: Visualization for Stability

INTRODUCTION: Visualization for stability is harnessing the power of the mind to improve your feeling of balance and stability. These exercises may be performed sitting, which promotes mental attention and physical well-being. Find a comfortable sitting posture with enough back support, and let's look at the advantages of visualizing for stability.

1. GROUNDING ROOT VISUALIZATION (5 MINS):

- Sit comfortably, with your back straight and your hands resting on your lap.

- Gently close your eyes, or lessen your stare if it seems more comfortable.

- To center yourself, take a few deep breaths.

- Imagine roots growing from the base of your spine into the earth, anchoring you like the roots of a robust tree.

- Imagine these roots stretching deep into the dirt to provide a solid foundation.

- As you inhale, envision pulling power and stability from the soil via these roots.

- Hold this imagery for a few seconds while feeling grounded and steady.

- Exhale slowly to relieve any tension.

- Repeat this Grounding Root Visualization for 5 minutes, allowing the feeling of stability to grow with each breath.

2. MOUNTAIN VISUALIZATION (5 MINS):

- Sit comfortably, back straight, hands on lap.

- Gently close your eyes, or lessen your stare if it seems more comfortable.

- To center yourself, take a few deep breaths.

- Visualize yourself as a beautiful mountain, lofty and powerful.

- Feel the mountain's strong, unchanging presence within you.

- Inhale deeply, imagining yourself absorbing the mountain's vitality and stability.

- Hold this vision for a few seconds, embracing the mountain's power and tenacity.

- Exhale softly to release any tension.

- Repeat this Mountain Visualization for 5 minutes, letting your sensation of stability to strengthen with each breath.

3. BALANCING BEAM VISUALIZATION (5 MINS):

- Sit comfortably, with your back straight and your hands resting on your lap.

- Gently close your eyes, or lessen your stare if it seems more comfortable.

- To center yourself, take a few deep breaths.

- Visualize a straight, thin balancing beam in front of you.

- Imagine yourself comfortably strolling down this beam while keeping perfect balance.

- As you inhale, consider the concentration and steadiness necessary to remain focused on the beam.

- Hold this vision for a few seconds to experience the synchronization and control.

- Exhale slowly to relieve any tension.

- Hold the Balancing Beam Visualization for 5 minutes, letting your sensation of stability to grow with each breath.

Conclusion:

Visualization for stability is an effective exercise that combines mental attention and bodily well-being. The Grounding Root Visualization, Mountain Visualization, and Balancing Beam Visualization all provide variants to improve your sense of stability. Regular practice of these exercises will result in enhanced balance, mental clarity, and a strong sense of grounding.

Day 21: Yoga Nidra for Deep Relaxation

INTRODUCTION: Yoga Nidra, commonly known as "yogic sleep," is a guided meditation that promotes profound relaxation. This exercise may be done while sitting comfortably, which promotes mental serenity and overall well-being. Find a quiet and comfortable area with enough back support, and let's look into the benefits of Yoga Nidra for deep relaxation.

1. BODY SCAN AND RELAXATION (15 MINS):

- Sit comfortably, with your back straight and your hands resting on your lap.

- Close your eyes lightly and allow your focus to shift within.

- Take a few deep breaths to relax into the present moment.

- Begin to direct your attention to different regions of your body, starting with your toes and gradually progressing to the top of your head.

- As you focus on each body area, intentionally relax and release whatever stress you may be carrying.

- Continue this body scan, allowing a sensation of calm to penetrate your whole being.

- The guided meditation will take you through each area of your body, encouraging profound relaxation.

- After the body scan, keep motionless and enjoy the feeling of tranquility for a few seconds.

- Gradually return your consciousness to the current moment, opening your eyes when you are ready.

2. BREATH AWARENESS AND CALMING (10 MINS):

- Sit comfortably, with your back straight and your hands resting on your lap.

- Close your eyes slightly, or soften your focus if it is more comfortable.

- Concentrate your attention on your breathing, noticing the natural pattern of intake and expiration.

- As you breathe in, quietly tell yourself, "I am aware of my inhale."

- As you breathe out, quietly tell yourself, "I am aware of my exhale."

- Allow your breath to flow freely, without attempting to regulate it.

- With each breath, let go of any ideas or distractions and focus your attention on the present now.

- The guided meditation will lead you through breathing exercises and relaxation methods.

- After the breath awareness practice, sit motionless and enjoy the peace for a few seconds.

- Gradually return your consciousness to the current moment, opening your eyes when you are ready.

3. GUIDED IMAGERY AND INNER PEACE (10 MINS):

- Sit comfortably, with your back straight and your hands resting on your lap.

- Close your eyes softly, allowing your mind to make room for guided images.

- The guided meditation will take you through a tranquil countryside, encouraging you to imagine pleasant sights.

- Engage all of your senses in this imagery: feel the warmth of the sun, hear the quiet rustle of leaves, and experience the peace around you.

- Allow the guided meditation to take you further into a state of inner serenity.

- After the guided visualization, keep motionless and enjoy the peace for a few seconds.

- Gradually return your consciousness to the current moment, opening your eyes when you are ready.

CONCLUSION: Yoga Nidra for deep relaxation is a restorative technique that blends guided meditation and mindful relaxation. The Body Scan and Relaxation, Breath Awareness and Calming, and Guided Imagery and Inner Peace activities all offer different ways to encourage deep relaxation. Practice these exercises on a daily basis to promote mental serenity, reduce stress, and boost general well-being. As with any new exercise, begin with short sessions and progressively expand as you feel more comfortable. As you continue your chair yoga journey, benefit from Yoga Nidra's profound relaxing effects.

DAY 15:

How did you feel after completing the seated cardio workout with marching, jumping jacks, and high knee taps? ----------------------

----

Did you notice any changes in your energy levels or overall well-being? --

----

DAY 16:

Reflect on your experience with the heel and toe taps. How did this exercise contribute to your awareness of ankle flexibility and lower leg strength? ---

----

Were you able to perform the movements comfortably? ----------

----

DAY 17:

After practicing the side leg raises, cross leg lifts, and leg circles, do you feel a difference in the strength and stability of your hips and thighs? --

----

How would you describe your experience with these seated exercises? ---

----

DAY 18:

Share your thoughts on the Chair Yoga Warrior Pose series. Did you find the seated variations of Warrior I, II, and III challenging or empowering? --

----

Notice any changes in your core strength and stability? -----------

----

DAY 19:

How did the Tree Pose with Support exercises impact your sense of balance and stability? ---

----

Describe your experience with the seated tree pose, supported leg extension, and seated ankle-to-knee pose. -------------------------

----

DAY 20:

Reflect on your practice of visualization for stability. Did the grounding root visualization, mountain visualization, and balancing beam visualization contribute to a sense of stability and calmness? Share your experience. -------------------------------------

----

Day 21:

After engaging in the Yoga Nidra for deep relaxation, how would you describe your mental and physical state? ------------------------

----

Did you notice any changes in your ability to unwind and find deep relaxation through guided meditation? ------------------------

----

Feel free to use these questions as a guide for your self-reflection, and take note of any observations or insights that arise during your chair yoga practice.

CHAPTER 6

Day 22: Seated Forward Bends

INTRODUCTION:

Welcome to Day 22 of the "28 Days Chair Yoga for Seniors." Seated forward bends are excellent for extending the spine and hamstrings while developing flexibility. This technique produces a slow release of tension and a feeling of peace. Let us begin the practice with comfort and ease.

1. PREPARATION (5 MINUTES)

- Sit comfortably on the edge of your strong chair, feet flat on the floor.

- Keep your back straight, shoulders relaxed, and hands resting on your thighs.

- Take a few deep breaths to help you center yourself and relax.

2. SEATED FORWARD BEND (10 MINS):

- Inhale and stretch your spine while gently activating your core.

- Exhale, bend at the hips, and lean forward from the waist.

- Depending on your comfort level, let your hands reach for the floor or grab the edges of your chair.

- Keep your back straight, and if it seems comfortable, slowly drop your chest towards your thighs.

- Maintain the pose for 20-30 seconds, inhaling deeply and feeling the stretch down your spine and the backs of your legs.

- Inhale as you gradually return to an upright position.

3. SEATED WIDE-LEG FORWARD BEND (10 MINS):

- Spread your legs and form a V shape with your feet.

- Inhale to stretch your spine, then exhale as you bend forward from your hips.

- Maintain a straight back and, if comfortable, place your hands on the floor or grip the chair.

- Feel the stretch in your inner thighs and spine.

- Hold the stance for 20-30 seconds while inhaling deeply.

- Inhale to softly rise back up.

4. SEATED TWIST (10 MINS):

- Sit with your spine upright and your legs uncrossed.

- Inhale to stretch your spine, then exhale and rotate to the right, resting your left hand on your right knee and your right hand on the back of the chair.

- Hold the twist for 15-20 seconds, experiencing the gradual movement of your spine.

- Inhale back into the middle and repeat the twist on the left side.

- Continue alternating sides for 5 minutes, feeling the renewing influence on your spine and body

Conclusion:

Seated forward bends are a wonderful way to improve flexibility and relieve stress in the back and legs. Remember to move lightly and within your body's limits. Today's practice may be both calming and energizing, improving your general wellbeing. As with any workout, listen to your body and reap the advantages of these sitting forward bends.

INTRODUCTION: Welcome to Day 23 of the 28 Days of Chair Yoga for Seniors. Gentle hip openers reduce tension and stiffness in the hips, increasing mobility and comfort. These exercises might help you become more flexible and make daily motions easier. Let's try three easy hip-opening movements together.

1. SEATED KNEE-TO-CHEST STRETCH (10 MINS):

- Sit comfortably on the edge of your chair, feet flat on the floor.

- Use the edges of your chair for support.

- Inhale deeply, and as you exhale, pull your right knee to your chest, holding it with both hands.

- Gently draw your knee closer to your chest until you feel a stretch in your hip and lower back.

- Hold the stretch for 20 to 30 seconds while breathing steadily.

- Release and move to the left leg, continuing the stretch for equal duration.

- Alternate between both legs for a total of 5 minutes, gradually increasing the strain with each repeat.

2. SEATED FIGURE-FOUR STRETCH (10 MINS):

- sit tall in your chair and place your feet flat on the floor.

- Lift your right foot and position the outside border of your right ankle against your left thigh, forming a figure-four with your legs.

- Keep your right knee softly pressed away from your body to protect the knee joint.

- If you're comfortable, gently press down on your right knee to feel a stretch in your right hip.

- Hold the stretch for 20-30 seconds while breathing steadily.

- Release and move to the left leg, continuing the stretch for equal duration.

- For 5 minutes, alternate between both legs, allowing the hips to relax and expand.

3. SEATED HIP CIRCLES (10 MINS):

- Sit comfortably on the edge of your chair, feet flat on the floor.

- Put your hands on your knees for support.

- Inhale deeply, and as you exhale, start making gently circular movements with your hips.

- Circle your hips clockwise 5 times, concentrating on smooth and controlled motions.

- Reverse the direction and circle your hips counterclockwise for 5 more times.

- Feel the gentle movement of your hip joints and the release of tension in the muscles around them.

- Continue for 5 minutes, allowing your hips to move freely.

CONCLUSION: Gentle hip openers provide a road to greater mobility and comfort in everyday activities. By including these exercises into your regimen, you may reduce stiffness and increase hip flexibility. Remember to walk gently and deliberately while respecting your body's requirements and limitations. Accept the relaxing effects of hip-opening exercises and appreciate the flexibility of mobility they provide in your life.

INTRODUCTION: Welcome to Day 24 of 28 Days of Chair Yoga for Seniors. Seated Cat-Cow stretches are a gentle and effective approach to improve spinal flexibility, promote mobility, and relieve tension. These workouts help you move more fluidly. Let's look at three types of Seated Cat-Cow stretches together.

1.SEATED CAT STRETCH (10 MINS):

- sitting comfortably on the edge of your chair with your feet flat on the floor.

- Put your hands on your knees for support.

- Inhale deeply and arch your back, elevating your chest to the ceiling.

- Tilt your pelvis forward and let your tummy sink gently.

- Experience a gentle stretch in your lower back and a pleasant opening in your chest.

- Hold this position for 20 to 30 seconds, concentrating on the stretch along your spine.

- Exhale gently and return to a neutral sitting position.

2. SEATED COW STRETCH (10 MINS):

- by exhaling and rounding your spine while tucking your chin towards your chest.

- Feel the stretch across your upper back and between your shoulder blades.

- Maintain this circular stance for 20-30 seconds while inhaling deeply.

- Inhale as you return to a neutral sitting posture.

- Repeat the Cat and Cow stretches for 5 minutes, alternating between the two postures in a fluid rhythm.

- Concentrate on the smooth articulation of your spine and the relaxing rhythm of your breathing.

3. SEATED CAT-COW FLOW (10 MINS):

- Sit comfortably, hands on knees.

- Inhale and arch your back into the Cat stretch.

- Exhale as you circle your spine for the Cow stretch.

- Continue to alternate between Cat and Cow stretches, synchronizing your breathing with each movement.

- Allow your spine's natural curvature to lead your action.

- Enjoy the rhythmic flow for 5 minutes, which will help you improve your spine's flexibility and mobility.

CONCLUSION: Seated Cat-Cow stretches are an enjoyable approach to stimulate the spine and increase flexibility. These movements gently massage your back muscles, relieving stress and improving your general sense of well-being. Embrace the flowing motions, move at your own pace, and enjoy the renewing impact these stretches have on your body.

INTRODUCTION: Welcome to Day 25 of 28 Days of Chair Yoga for Seniors. A full-body stretch regimen is an excellent approach to increase flexibility, improve circulation, and energize your body. Today, we'll look at three restorative stretches that target diverse muscle areas. Let's go on a trip to reenergize your complete body.

1. SEATED NECK-TO-TOE STRETCH (15 MINS):

- Begin by sitting comfortably on the edge of your chair, feet flat on the floor.

- Inhale deeply, raising your arms aloft and interlacing your fingers.

- As you exhale, gently lean to one side, causing a lateral stretch in your torso.

- Hold the stretch for 20-30 seconds and feel the elongation on the other side.

- Inhale back into the center, then exhale as you lean to the opposite side.

- Repeat this side-to-side motion for 5 minutes, letting your breath lead the movement.

- This stretch focuses on the sides of your body and promotes spinal flexibility.

2. SEATED SPINAL TWIST (15 MINS):

- Sit tall on your chair, with your feet firmly planted on the floor.

- Inhale deeply, then exhale while twisting your upper body to the right, resting your left hand on the outside of your right knee and your right hand on the back of the chair.

- Hold the twist for 20-30 seconds, experiencing a slight rotation of your spine.

- Inhale back into the center, then exhale as you rotate to the left, repeating the stretch on the other side.

- Continue alternating right and left twists for 5 minutes.

- This stretch increases spinal flexibility and creates a sense of well-being.

3. FULL BODY EXTENSION (15 MINS):

- sit comfortably with your back straight and feet flat on the floor.

- Inhale deeply and extend your arms upwards, interlacing your fingers.

- Exhale while leaning slightly forward, stretching your arms in front of you and reaching for your toes.

- Hold the stretch for 20-30 seconds to feel a mild stretch around your spine, hamstrings, and shoulders.

- Inhale as you return to an upright position.

- Repeat the forward extension for 5 minutes, allowing the breath to guide your movement.

- This stretch targets the entire back, hamstrings, and shoulders, resulting in a full-body stretch.

CONCLUSION: A full-body stretch regimen promotes overall flexibility and regeneration. These exercises increase suppleness in many muscle areas, leaving you feeling refreshed and energized. As usual, move at your own pace, listen to your body, and enjoy the renewing effects these stretches provide for your complete self. Enjoy the process of nurturing your body with this full-body stretch practice.

Day 26: Chair Yoga Sun Salutations

INTRODUCTION: Welcome to Day 26 of the 28 Days Chair Yoga for Seniors. Chair Yoga Sun Salutations promote energy, awareness, and full-body participation. This sequence is intended to energize your body, increase circulation, and promote overall wellness. Let us go on this revitalizing trip together.

1. SEATED MOUNTAIN POSE (10 MINS):

- Start by sitting comfortably on the edge of your chair, feet flat on the floor.

- Inhale deeply while raising your arms upwards, palms facing each other.

- Engage your core and extend upwards to lengthen your spine.

- Maintain the stretch for 20-30 seconds, experiencing the extension throughout your body.

- Exhale and lower your hands to your heart center.

- This position provides a solid foundation and creates a thoughtful tone for the Sun Salutation.

2. SEATED FORWARD FOLD (10 MINS):

- Inhale, raising your arms overhead once again.

- Exhale and bend at the hips, leaning forward with a straight spine.

- Let your hands reach toward the floor or grab the edges of your chair.

- Hold the stretch for 20-30 seconds until you feel a mild relaxation in your spine and hamstrings.

- Inhale to get back to an upright position.

- This forward fold stretches the spine and prepares you for the flowing sequence.

3. SEATED SUN SALUTATION FLOW (20 MINS):

- Inhale and raise your arms upwards.

- Exhale and lower your hands to your heart in prayer position.

- Inhale, stretching your arms forth and upward while gently arching your back.

- Exhale and bend at the hips, then go into a sitting forward fold.

- Inhale and return to an upright position, arms aloft.

- Exhale and bring your hands back to your heart.

- Continue this flowing sequence for 10 minutes, synchronizing your breathing with each movement.

- Experience the revitalizing benefits of this dynamic Sun Salutation Flow.

CONCLUSION:

Chair Yoga. Sun Salutations are a lively and easy method to utilize your entire body. The flowing routine encourages flexibility, circulation, and a feeling of vibrancy. As you progress through each posture, concentrate on the rhythm of your breathing and the subtle activation of your muscles. Accept the energizing advantages of Sun Salutations and let the energy flow through your body, leaving you feeling rejuvenated and energized. Enjoy the journey of movement and awareness in this Sun Salutation exercise.

INTRODUCTION: Welcome to day 27 of 28 Days of Chair Yoga for Seniors. Joint mobility exercises are essential for preserving flexibility, avoiding stiffness, and improving general joint health. Today, we'll look at three moderate yet effective joint mobility exercises for increasing range of motion in specific locations. Let us prioritize the health of your joints together.

1. NECK CIRCLES (10 MINS):

- Sit comfortably on the edge of your chair, back straight.

- Inhale and slowly lower your chin to your chest.

- Exhale, then gently swivel your head to the right, bringing your ear near your right shoulder.

- Inhale and continue in a circular motion, pulling your head back, then exhale as you circle to the left.

- Continue in a calm and controlled circular motion for 5 minutes.

- Reverse the direction and continue for another 5 minutes.

- This exercise increases neck flexibility and mobility, which relieves tension and improves circulation.

2. SHOULDER ROLLS (10 MINS):

- Sit comfortably, with your feet flat on the floor.

- Inhale as you raise both shoulders to your ears.

- Exhale, then move your shoulders backward in a circular motion, pressing the shoulder blades together.

- Continue the circular motion for 5 minutes while breathing steadily.

- Roll your shoulders forward for another 5 minutes, then reverse the direction.

- This exercise improves shoulder mobility, decreases stiffness, and increases blood flow to the upper body.

3. ANKLE ALPHABET (15 MINS):

- Sit upright with feet flat on the ground.

- Lift your right foot slightly off the ground and spin your ankle to form the letters of the alphabet in the air.

- Use your right foot to go slowly and methodically through the whole alphabet.

- Lower your right foot and then repeat the exercise with your left.

- Continue to alternate between both feet for a total of 15 minutes.

- Ankle alphabet exercises are great for keeping the ankles flexible, boosting circulation, and reducing stiffness.

CONCLUSION:

Joint mobility exercises are critical for maintaining flexibility and avoiding stiffness in certain parts of the body. Including these mild motions in your regimen will help with overall joint health, allowing you to move more easily and freely.

Day 28: Celebration and Reflection

INTRODUCTION: Congratulations on Day 28 of 28 Days of Chair Yoga for Seniors! Today is a day to celebrate and contemplate. We'll do three important exercises to recognize your accomplishments, express thanks, and reflect on your journey. Let us recognize your effort and the beneficial influence it has had on your well-being.

1. GRATITUDE MEDITATION (15 MINS):

- Find a quiet, comfortable place to sit on the edge of your chair, feet flat on the ground.

- To find your core, close your eyes and take a few deep breaths.

- Begin by reflecting on the previous 28 days and appreciating your efforts to improve your well-being.

- Change your emphasis to things you are grateful for in your life, whether they are little or deep.

- With each breath, say quietly, "I am grateful for..."

- With each breath, imagine the things you're grateful for and feel the wonderful emotions that come with them.

- Continue this exercise for 15 minutes, expressing appreciation for the journey and the wonderful improvements that have occurred.

2. CHAIR YOGA FLOW REVIEW (10 MINS):

- Sit comfortably in your chair and focus on your breath.

- Review some of the most important chair yoga postures and sequences you've learned over the last 28 days.

- Practice a mild chair yoga sequence that incorporates your favorite postures and stretches.

- Move attentively, paying attention to your body's feelings and breath.

- Spend 10 minutes doing a tailored chair yoga session to celebrate your increased flexibility and overall well-being.

3. JOURNALING AND REFLECTION (15 MINS):

- Get out a diary or a piece of paper and a pen.

- Reflect on your chair yoga experience, including how you felt on Day 1, the problems you encountered, and the development you've made.

- Record any discoveries, realizations, or beneficial changes you've seen in your body and mind.

- Consider how chair yoga has changed your everyday life and if you wish to continue with any specific practices.

- Spend 15 minutes journaling and thinking on your transforming experience.

CONCLUSION:

As you finish "28 Days Chair Yoga for Seniors," take a minute to appreciate your dedication to wellness and the good improvements you've made. The gratitude meditation, chair yoga flow review, and writing activities are effective ways to recognize your accomplishments and reflect on your personal development. Your commitment to this trip is admirable, and the benefits will undoubtedly be seen in many areas of your life. Celebrate your accomplishment and incorporate the nourishing benefits of chair yoga into your continuing wellness path. Thank you for participating in this transformational experience!

DAY 22:

How did the seated forward bends make you feel physically and emotionally today? --

----

DAY 23:

Did you notice any changes in your hip mobility after engaging in the gentle hip openers today? --

----

DAY 24:

How did the seated Cat-Cow stretches contribute to your sense of relaxation and flexibility? --

----

DAY 25:

What was your favorite part of the full body stretch routine, and how did it make you feel overall? ------------------------------------

----

DAY 26:

How did practicing chair yoga sun salutations impact your energy levels and overall mood? --

----

DAY 27:

Which joint mobility exercise did you find most beneficial for your body, and why? ---

----

DAY 28:

As you reflect on the entire chair yoga journey, what positive changes have you observed in your physical and mental well-being? --

----

Feel free to use these questions as a guide for personal reflection and self-assessment. They are designed to help you understand and appreciate the progress and benefits you've experienced throughout the 28 days of chair yoga.

CONCLUSION

As we conclude our journey through 28 Days Chair Yoga challenge for Seniors, it's essential to reflect on the transformative experiences we've shared. Throughout these 28 days, we've explored the gentle yet profound practice of chair yoga, nurturing our bodies, minds, and spirits.

From the foundational poses to the flowing sequences, each day has offered an opportunity to connect with ourselves on a deeper level, fostering a sense of well-being and vitality. We've celebrated moments of triumph and navigated challenges with grace, recognizing that every breath and movement is a step towards greater health and harmony.

Through the practice of chair yoga, we've discovered the power of mindfulness, the importance of self-care, and the resilience of the human spirit. We've cultivated strength, flexibility, and inner peace, embracing the beauty of aging with grace and gratitude.

As we bid farewell to these 28 days, let us carry the lessons learned and the wisdom gained into our daily lives. Let us continue to prioritize our health and wellness, honoring our bodies and minds with compassion and kindness.

May the gentle rhythms of chair yoga accompany us on our journey forward, serving as a source of inspiration and rejuvenation. Let us remember that the path to well-being is not a destination but a continuous journey—one that we embark on with courage, curiosity, and an open heart.

Thank you for joining me on this transformative adventure. May your days be filled with joy, vitality, and the enduring spirit of chair yoga.